The Pegan Diet Food

A Healthy Way To Live Longer

Louis F. Morris

Contents

Chapter 1

WHAT MAKES THIS DIET DIFFERENT THAN OTHER FAMOUS DIETS?

The Pegan diet is a hybrid of many diets. It is, nonetheless, unique among all of them. Let's take a look at how a Pegan diet varies from other popular eating plans:

Paleo

A paleo diet, by definition, is based on the belief that our bodies function best when we eat as our forefathers did. Nuts and seeds, healthy oils, organic items, veggies, and meat were all included in this diet in small amounts. Nothing false, dairy products, beans, potatoes, cereals (excluding maize), or processed food variations were allowed. There would be no agricultural development of crops and cereals, and the meat eaten would be often thin. Grass-fed and natural foods would make up the majority of the diet in most cases.

A Pegan diet, on the other hand, combines the finest aspects of both paleo and vegetarian diets. As a result, you eat fewer servings of solid oils, natural goods, veggies, and meats, and avoid added sugars, gluten, and dairy.

One of the most common misconceptions about the paleo diet is that it is primarily a meat-based diet. A mountain man's diet consisting only of meat would have been unthinkable. It's tough to bring down massive beasts, and chasing them down would take a long time.

As a result, as a supplement, our forefathers started consuming nuts, veggies, natural goods, and vegetables.

The similarities between a Pegan and a paleo diet, however, end here. Getting in shape on a paleo diet is much more difficult since you are still consuming gluten-free grains such as rice, maize, and oats, which contribute a lot of extra calories. You don't eat more than a single serving of gluten on the Pegan diet.

Vegan

A vegan diet is 100 percent plant-based, but a Pegan diet must be at least 75 percent plant-based. A vegan diet is a style of life that avoids using any animal-based products for clothing, food, or other uses. As a result, a vegan diet excludes dairy, eggs, and meats from the diet.

People choose to eat vegetarian for a variety of reasons, ranging from environmental concerns to moral concerns. They may, however, be motivated by a desire to enhance one's health.

A Pegan diet, on the other hand, is almost vegetarian. A Pegan diet includes creature-based side dishes rather than things cultivated from the earth. Everything vegetarian makes up the foundation of this diet.

Dairy products are also avoided on a Pegan diet.

A vegan diet is extremely similar to a Pegan diet, as we can see from the above. A vegan diet, on the other hand, forbids the consumption of meat, poultry, and fish. Vegans also exclude other animal-based items such as honey and eggs, as well as any other products containing animal by-products such as leather, wool, cosmetics, and so on, from their lives and diets. Animal-based goods are permitted on a Pegan diet, but only 25% of your plate must be made up of them; the remaining 75% must be made up of plant-based foods.

Vegetarian

For a variety of reasons, some people may choose to follow a plant-based diet rather than eating meat. A vegetarian loving diet, by definition, is a way of eating that excludes any animal-based foods such as eggs, dairy, fish, chicken, and meat. A vegan diet, on the other hand, excludes all animal products such as fish, poultry, and meat. They are, however, allowed to eat a limited number of animal-based products, such as dairy.

4   THE PEGAN DIET FOOD

There are a lot of similarities between a vegetable lover's diet and the Pegan diet. Plant-based foods are included in both types of diets, for example.

The likenesses, however, stop here. You are not allowed to consume any dairy products, such as margarine or milk, while on the Pegan diet.

Furthermore, regardless of whether the grains are whole or refined, you are not authorized to polish them off.

Unlike the Pegan diet, you are also not allowed to consume meat, eggs, or meat of any type. However, it is also dependent on the kind of vegan diet that you follow. A flexitarian diet, often known as a semi-vegetarian diet, allows you to consume dairy products and eggs while also allowing you to consume small amounts of fish, chicken, and meat. Then there's the Pescatarian diet, which allows you to eat seafood, fish, dairy products, and eggs but prohibits you from eating chicken or beef.

Chapter 2

RULES FOR A PEGAN DIET IN CHAPTER 2

The Pegan diet is influenced by two prominent diets: the paleo and vegan diets, as previously stated. The goal of this diet, according to Dr. Hyman, is to promote maximum health by regulating blood sugar levels and reducing inflammation.

inflammation is reduced The following are some of the rules to follow while following a Pegan diet:

Vegetables and fruits that are in season should be chosen.

Leafy vegetables must account for 75% of your plate on a Pegan diet. They should, in fact, be a regular part of your diet. They are rich in minerals and nutrients that keep you healthy and protect you from sickness.

For a more active, healthy, normal, and adaptable way of living, most people would benefit from consuming more veggies and organiC products. Vegetables and organic goods provide a variety of minerals and nutrients that are beneficial to your health, such as folic acid, phosphorus, zinc, magnesium, and other vitamins and minerals such as E, C, A (beta-carotene), and others.

Sugar, salt, and fat are all in short supply in fruits and vegetables. They're high in dietary fiber and low in calories. You will really desire to maintain a healthy weight and reduce stoutness with the help of natural items. You'll also lower your blood pressure and cholesterol levels.

Strong phytochemicals are found in fruits and vegetables, which help to protect your overall health. Phytochemicals are mostly associated with color, which means that vegetables and natural products with different tones, such as white, blue-purple, red, yellow-orange, and green, each have their own unique blend of vitamins and phytochemicals that work together to promote good health. White vegetables such as cauliflower, for example, include sulforaphane, which may help protect against some types of malignancies; green vegetables such as kale and spinach, on the other hand, contain zeaxanthin and lutein, which protect against age-related medical issues such as eye illnesses. Later in this part, we'll go into more detail on the Rainbow diet.

It is vital to eat a variety of soil-based products if you want to increase your supplement intake. You may try buying green foods according to the seasons; this is nature's way of ensuring that your body receives a healthy mix of plant synthetics and nutrients. You may, on the other hand, opt to buy a variety of soil items and experiment with different recipes.

It is critical to focus on quality.

Genuine food sources are foods that are rich in nutrients, free of compound added ingredients, and typically natural, and are associated with a Pegan diet. In general, these are the kinds of foods that early humans ate. In the twentieth century, however, handled food variety grew well-known and shifted dramatically toward ready-to-eat meals. While processed foods are convenient and quick, they are also harmful to human health. Indeed, one of the most important things you can do for your body to maintain a high-quality life and wonderful wellness is to consume authentic, high-quality food sources. Your overall health will be influenced by the kind of foods you consume.

The nature of the food variety and fixes are critical to the success of any diet. In essence, the nature of the food sources for a Pegan diet should be nothing short of amazing. A typical Pegan dish requires 2-3 fresh cups of produce, with vibrant, drab greens and other non-boring veggies included. It's also a good idea to mix it up with lovely veggies and organic goods to create the most nutritious thickness. Because a Pegan diet places a premium on quality, it is recommended that you use natural and privately made foods wherever feasible.

A few creature-based things are also included in a Pegan's diet. These meals, in any event, are meant to be served as a complement to the plant-based main courses. Eggs, poultry, and red meat should all be farmed in a humane manner or be grass-fed. The fish should be caught in the wild and should have less mercury.

Pegan diets also include omega-3 unsaturated fats, which are recognized to be powerful anti-inflammatory agents. Fish, such as herring, mackerel, anchovies, sardines, and salmon, should be wild-caught grease fishes.

75 percent of your total food should be made up of plant foods.

Consume the Full Spectrum

Experts advise that you 'consume the rainbow' for the healthiest admittance possible. This implies that you consume bright veggies and organic goods, as previously said. These are beneficial to the body in several ways.

Shades, also known as phytonutrients, may be found in plants in numerous forms. They get a diverse range of tones from these phytonutrients. Vegetables and organic items of various hues and textures have long been linked to certain health benefits and supplements. While eating a lot of leafy greens is good, it's also important to focus on eating a variety of colored plants to increase your intake of various vitamins that will benefit every aspect of your overall health.

While phytonutrients offer several benefits, conducting randomized controlled trials is challenging - as a result, experts have compiled their research on admissions and disease risk in light of the general population. According to these studies, eating vibrant veggies and natural goods offers several benefits and almost no drawbacks. You'll get a variety of phytochemicals, minerals, and vitamins by including shade in your Pegan diet.

Let's have a look at a few different tones and see how they might help you feel better: Red

Grapefruit, pink guava, watermelon, tomato, and others are examples of fruits and vegetables. The principal phytonutrient is Lycopene is a kind of antioxidant that is found in tomatoes (Vitamin A family)

Vitamins and minerals not mentioned above: K1 is a kind of vitamin that helps the body to

Potassium Folate Vitamin C Vitamin C Vitamin C Vitamin C Vitamin C Vitamin C Vitamin C Vitamin C

Benefits to your health: Reduces your chances of developing some malignancies.

Skin damage from the sun should be minimized.

Heart health is improved

Orange and yellow are two complementary colors.

Squash, pumpkin, bananas, tangerines, pineapple, carrots, yellow peppers, and other fruits and vegetables are among the fruits and vegetables.

The principal phytonutrient is Carotenoids are a kind of antioxidant that is found in plants (Vitamin A family) Vitamins and minerals not mentioned above:

C is a powerful antioxidant.

Potassium Vitamin A is a powerful antioxidant that helps the body Fiber rich in folate

Cancer risks are reduced as a result of using this supplement.

Eye health is aided

Heart health is improved

Green spices, Brussel sprouts, green cabbage, asparagus, avocados, broccoli, kale, spinach, and other green fruits and vegetables are examples.

In salad greens, carotenoids and chlorophyll are abundant, whereas cruciferous greens include glucosinolates, isothiocyanates, and indoles (cabbage, broccoli)

Vitamin K1 is an example of a mineral or vitamin that is not found in the body.

Vitamin A is a powerful antioxidant that helps the body

Potassium

Fiber Fiber Magnesium Folate Magnesium Folate Magnesium Folate Magn

Benefits to your health: Reduces your chance of heart disease and cancer.

Antioxidant

Anti-inflammatory

Gluten-free diet

The labels "gluten-free" and "dairy-free" have become more popular.

during the last several years Many people who aren't gluten intolerant have discovered ways to manage chronic illnesses, dietary inequity, and annoyance. Dairy and gluten are common allergies that may result in a variety of medical problems.

Gluten, also known as prolamin, is a kind of protein present in grains such as rye, barley, and wheat. Because gluten is known to be flexible, it is usually referred to as "magic" that binds prepared foods. Gluten causes inflammation in the body in a variety of ways. This is due to the fact that it includes substantial amounts of supplement enemies, which are proteins present in certain plants.

These supplement foes are bad for the body since they prevent food from being properly digested and absorbed in the stomach, resulting in inflammation.

Gluten consumption also causes the body to release zonulin. Zonulin is a kind of protein that regulates how the junctions in the stomach lining open and close. Our stomach is very permeable, allowing good substances to enter the circulatory system while harmful substances are stored in the stomach for eventual elimination.

When you finish zonulin, it slows the stomach's porousness and keeps the junctions open.

Sheep's milk, goat's milk, cow's milk, and even camel's milk are all examples of dairy products. Margarine, cheddar, kefir, yogurt, and cream are just a few examples of dairy-based products. Dairy is classified as a difficult-to-process allergic food that causes inflammation.

Lactose bias, for example, is a disease caused by dairy consumption. Lactose is a sugar present in milk that needs the synthesis of the chemical lactase in order for the body to metabolize it. When we are young, our bodies produce this protein, but as we become older, we lose this ability. Lactose intolerance affects around 65 percent of adults worldwide.

Casein, particularly A1 casein, is a protein found in dairy products that might cause problems with safe framework capacity and digestion. If lactose and A1 casein are bothering your stomach, look for alternate dairy options. Goat milk, for example, has a lower lactose content than cow milk.

Vegetable oils aren't good for you.

Vegetable oils are bad for your health and for the environment, which few people are aware of. Oils extracted from seeds such as nut, safflower, sunflower, maize, soybean, and rapeseed will be known as vegetable oils (canola oil). These vegetable oils are extracted in an artificial manner, unlike olive and coconut oils, which are separated by squeezing.

Apart from the commonly held belief that these oils are bad for you because they contain omega-3 unsaturated fats and monounsaturated fats, these oils are often marketed as healthy.

These bogus health claims will almost always be targeted by advancements. Regardless, this does not constitute a complete image arrangement.

The truth is that vegetable oils are abundant in polyunsaturated fats (PUFAs), but the human body is mostly monounsaturated and saturated fats. Fat is needed for hormone synthesis as well as cell regeneration. PUFAs, on the other hand, are very unstable and easily oxidized. As a result, cell mutation and inflammation are possible outcomes. Other forms of cardiac disorders have been connected to oxidation.

Omega-3 fatty acids, as we all know, are very beneficial to our health. The ratio of omega-3 to omega-6 acids, on the other hand, is critical for overall health.

Many omega-6 fatty acids are found in vegetable oils. The oxidation of these acids is quite fast. Omega-3 fatty acids, on the other hand, have been demonstrated to lower inflammation and protect against cancer. Different sorts of malignancies and other health issues have been related to unbalanced amounts of both types of acids.

Aside from the abnormally high quantities of omega-6 fatty acids and polyunsaturated fats, these vegetable oils also include chemicals, pesticides, and industrial additives. BHT and BHA are natural antioxidants that keep food from deteriorating too soon. However, research has shown that they may develop cancer-causing chemicals in the body. Finally, vegetable oil has been related to kidney and liver damage, as well as behavioral disorders, infertility, and immune system problems.

Gluten-free grains should be avoided.

Gluten is a naturally occurring protein present in grains such as rye, barley, and wheat, as previously discussed. This material has a flexible texture that helps to keep the meal together. Triticale, einkorn, Khorasan wheat, graham, farro, farina, semolina, emmer, durum, spelt, and wheat berries are only a few examples of gluten-containing grains. While oats are natively gluten-free, cross-contamination occurs when they are prepared with the grains previously mentioned. Modified food starch and soy sauce are two less apparent gluten-containing options.

The thing that is not great about gluten is that it can cause side effects in some people. People react to gluten differently– when the body recognizes it as a toxin, it will deploy the immune cells to attack it. If you are sensitive to gluten and consume it accidentally, it will result in inflammation. The side effects can range from mild effects like diarrhea, alternating constipation, bloating, and Irritable bowel syndrome, malnutrition, and unintentional weight loss are all symptoms of fatigue that can range from mild to severe.

Celiac disease affects one out of every 113 Americans, according to estimates; celiac disease patients have a higher risk of anemia and osteoporosis, according to research. Other health issues, such as nerve disorders, infertility, and even cancer, can result as a result of this.

The good news is that by eliminating gluten from your diet, you can reverse the damage. Celiac disease is frequently treated by following a gluten-free diet. Following a gluten-free diet, on the other hand, is not easy; you may need to seek advice from a registered dietician to learn which foods contain gluten and how to obtain other nutrients from gluten-free alternatives.

In a nutshell, a gluten-free diet involves avoiding gluten-containing foods. However, iron, magnesium, and vitamins are all present in most gluten-free whole grains. As a result, it's critical that you replenish the nutrients you've been missing. Consider poultry, eggs, fish, nuts, and whole fruits and vegetables, which are naturally gluten-free.

PREPARE TO GO PEGAN IN CHAPTER 3

People are starting the Pegan diet in droves these days; it's the latest fad in dieting. Is it possible for you to consume animal products? Yes, but only if you don't go overboard.

How about ingredients that have been processed? Only a few are suitable for consumption. This diet focuses on whole foods, so you'll be eating plenty of fresh fruits and vegetables.

The Pegan diet is a hybrid of the vegan and paleo diets, based on the belief that whole foods can help you achieve optimal health by lowering inflammation and balancing blood sugar levels.

Combining vegan and paleo diets may appear to be contradictory or strange at first glance. You can be certain that it isn't the case. Instead, think of it as a middle ground that combines the best aspects of both diets.

Meal planning is straightforward at its core. Pegan diet recipes include small amounts of high-quality animal-based proteins, as well as plenty of healthy fat, fruits, and vegetables, as previously mentioned.

You must also avoid legumes (peanuts, lentils, peas, and beans), grains, and dairy products.

Vegan and paleo diets both follow the same program's tenets:

Olive oil, seeds, nuts, avocados, and omega-3 fatty acids are all good sources of good fats.

Pesticides aren't used as much as they used to be. Organic, hormone-free, antibiotic-free, and non-GMO foods are just a few of the options. Chemical-free environment: There are no MSG, dyes, artificial sweeteners, or other additives in this product.

Look for deep and vibrant colors in your vegetables and fruits; the more variety, the better.

Low glycemic index: Refined carbohydrates, flour, and sugar are all low on the glycemic index scale. If you choose the Pegan diet, you will benefit from the following:

Sugary foods should be consumed in moderation; they can be enjoyed as a treat on rare occasions.

Legumes, grains, and dairy products should be avoided at all costs.

Seeds and nuts are high in protein and can help you avoid diabetes and heart disease.

Vegetables should account for approximately 75% of your daily calories.

Consume healthy fats such as omega-3 fatty acids, seeds, olive oil, nuts, and avocados; avoid soy and vegetable oils.

Consume low-glycemic-index foods, such as sardines, olive oil, seeds, nuts, and avocados, to get more fats and proteins.

Controversy

Pegan recipes and diet have grown in popularity significantly since 2014. In 2021, for example, Pinterest searches for "eating Pegan" increased by 337 percent. This diet, on the other hand, has generated a lot of debate.

Experts suggested, for example, that the general parameters of this diet are simply combining two opposing diet ideologies into a new type of diet. However, they believe that the majority of the Pegan diet's restrictions are time-consuming, expensive, and unnecessary. According to these nutritional and dietary experts, restricting legumes, for example, could pose a problem. Legumes are low-fat, high-fiber, and a rich source of protein, according to studies, and are an important part of the popular Mediterranean diet.

Furthermore, legumes have been linked to a variety of health benefits, including the prevention of cardiovascular disease, cancer, and other illnesses.

Recommendations

While the Pegan diet has sparked some debate, it has also received a lot of praise. Local and fresh is great, according to experts; however, most of these experts agree with Dr. Hyman that animal-based products should be served as a side dish rather than the main course. Increased consumption of vegetables, fruits, and seafood is also a popular suggestion among scientists.

Others have agreed that a Pegan diet has many advantages; for example, the emphasis on omega-3 fatty acids, fruits, and vegetables, as well as the factor of adequate protein, are all major advantages. In the end, a Pegan diet could be beneficial to your health. You will, however, be bound by some limitations. The Pegan diet will begin to have a beneficial effect on your body if you are able to do so.

Shopping List for Pegan

Now that you know what you're getting yourself into, here are a few items that must be on your shopping list:

Tomatoes, peas, carrots, broccoli, mushrooms, leeks, eggplant, peppers, cauliflower, Brussel sprouts, greens (turnip, mustard, collard, etc.), bamboo shoots, and other vegetables with a low glycemic index or starch content should all be included in your diet.

Fruits: Look for fruits with a low starch or glycemic index, similar to vegetables; these include pineapple, mangoes, pears, citrus fruits, dark berries, cherries, apples, oranges, watermelons, and so on. Fruits with a lot of water in them are the best to buy.

You can eat whole eggs, chicken, beef, pork, venison, and other animal proteins as long as the meat is grass-fed and sustainably sourced. Seafood, such as shrimp and salmon, are also acceptable.

Healthy Fats: A Pegan diet requires minimally processed fats from specific sources such as nuts (except peanuts), seeds (except processed seed oils), coconut oil (unrefined), olives, and avocados (ensure avocado and olive oil are coldpressed), as well as omega-3 fatty acids (ensure the fish has low mercury content).

Oils and butters: You won't be able to eat conventional butter because you can't eat dairy products. Vegan butter, mashed avocado, and other alternatives to butter exist. Sesame oil, olive oil, and other oils, on the other hand, are examples of oils. Vegetable oils should not be consumed.

Hemp, almond, soy, cashew, hazelnut, and oat are all excellent dairy substitutes for a Pegan diet.

Natural sugars such as vanilla, dates, honey, coconut sugar, and maple syrup can be included in your diet as sweeteners.

Except for peanuts, most nuts and seeds, such as almonds and walnuts, can be eaten. Chia, pumpkin, and flax seeds are some of the healthiest seeds available.

While legumes are generally discouraged in the Pegan diet, gluten-free whole legumes are allowed in limited quantities. No more than 75 grams of sugar per day should be consumed. Pinto beans, black beans, chickpeas, and lentils are just a few of the many examples.

Miscellaneous: You can use a variety of miscellaneous ingredients as long as they are natural and low in glycemic index.

Consumption of starchy foods should be limited. Even if you eat starch, make sure it comes from healthy sources. Baking products: Make sure the ingredients are refined sugar-free and gluten-free when making baking products. Black rice, quinoa, oats, black beans, and chickpeas can all be added to the mix.

Supplements: Supplements such as Vitamin D3 and omega-3 fatty acids can be used as part of a Pegan diet. Vitamin B12 is another option.

Pegan Meal Plan for One Week

A Pegan diet focuses on fruits and vegetables, but it also includes seeds, nuts, fish, and sustainably raised meats. Gluten-free grains and legumes can also be used in moderation. Here's a week-long menu plan:

Monday

Breakfast: Make a vegetable omelet and serve it with a simple green salad drizzled in olive oil.

Lunch: A simple salad with avocado, strawberries, and chickpeas is an excellent choice.

Wednesday Thursday Friday Saturday Tuesday Wednesday Thursday

Dinner ideas include wild salmon patties with lemon vinaigrette, steamed broccoli, and roasted carrots.

Breakfast: A sweet potato toast with lemon vinaigrette, pumpkin seeds, and sliced avocado is a simple way to start the day.

Make a Bento box for lunch with blackberries, fermented pickles, raw vegetable sticks, sliced turkey, and boiled eggs.

Dinner: Bring the day to a close with a vegetable stir-fry featuring black beans, tomato, bell pepper, onions, and cashews.

Breakfast: A green smoothie made with hemp seeds, almond butter, kale, and apple is a healthy and simple way to start your day.

Lunch: An easy lunch made with leftover vegetable stir-fry from Tuesday. Dinner: Vegetable kebabs, grilled shrimp, and black rice pilaf are among the options for a filling meal.

Breakfast: Chia seed and coconut pudding with fresh blueberries and walnuts is the best option for this day's breakfast.

Lunch: A mixed green salad with cider vinaigrette, grilled chicken, cucumber, and avocado is a good choice for today's lunch. Dinner: A delectable roasted beet salad with sliced almonds, Brussel sprouts, and pumpkin seeds is a delicious option.

Breakfast: A good start for breakfast is braised greens, kimchi, and fried eggs. Lunch: Serve vegetable stew with lentils and sliced cantaloupe as a side dish.

Dinner: Finish off the weekend with a salad featuring grass-fed beef strips, guacamole, jicama, and radishes.

Overnight oats, berries, walnuts, chia seeds, and cashew milk are a delicious way to start your Saturdays.

Lunch: Vegetable stew from the day before and lentils. Dinner: Serve roasted pork loin with quinoa, greens, and steamed vegetables as part of a special Saturday night dinner.

Breakfast: Make a simple vegetable omelet and a green salad for a lazy Sunday breakfast.

Lunch: Try the salad rolls with orange slices and cashew cream sauce, which are Thai-styled.

Finish the week with pork loin and vegetables from the night before.

PEGAN COOKING (CHAPTER 4)

Here are a few delicious Pegan-friendly recipes:

Breakfast

1. Avocado and Zucchini Baked Eggs

This dish is perfect if you want something savory instead of sweet.

You've made the ideal choice. Furthermore, this is a light dish. This dish is high in protein and fat, and it's a great way to start your day. It's a filling and flavorful vegetarian breakfast. This dish is healthy, quick to prepare, gluten-free, and Pegan-friendly, and it's perfect for the whole family.

Ingredients

Spray anti-stick

3 spiralized zucchini 2 tablespoons black pepper, Kosher salt, extra-virgin olive oil

Garnish with four large eggs, four red pepper flakes, and fresh basil 2 thinly sliced avocados, halved

Directions for Making Food

Preheat the oven to 350 degrees Fahrenheit. Using non-stick spray, lightly grease a baking sheet.

Toss the zucchini noodles and olive oil in a large mixing bowl until they are thoroughly combined. Add pepper and salt to taste to the mixture.

Divide the noodles into four equal parts and place them on a baking sheet in a nest shape.

Bake the dish until the eggs are set, or until the timer goes off at 11 minutes.

Add salt and pepper to taste to the dish. For garnish, you can use basil and red pepper flakes. Avocado slices can be added to the mix as well.

Chapter 4

Vegan Frittata with Vegetables

If you're looking for an inexpensive and quick vegan meal, the vegan frittata is the dish to make. Breakfast, lunch, or dinner, this delectable dish is a must-try.

Frittatas are an Italian dish. It can be made with any vegetable and eggs of your choice. A flavorful tofu-based 'egg' mixture will be used in this vegan frittata, along with a variety of other vegetables.

You'll be hard pressed to find someone who dislikes frittata, regardless of when you prepare it or eat it. Although this vegan frittata does not resemble the egg version, it is still high in protein and fiber and low in cholesterol, making it an excellent vegan dish.

This filling and flavorful tofu frittata is made with tofu. While it isn't necessary, a drizzle of sriracha or avocado on top for added heat is optional. You can make this vegan dish with products that are about to expire in your fridge.

Ingredients

Skinned or un-skinned potatoes Onions Peppers (bell) Zucchini Squash, bright yellow Garlic

Silken tofu that hasn't been pressed organically Non-dairy milk, unsweetened organic corn starch Yeast for food

Dijon, whole grain mustard, or a combination of the two Basil, thyme, or tarragon Turmeric

Powdered garlic salt and black pepper flakes de pimento

Directions for Making Food

Preheat oven to 375 degrees Fahrenheit.

In a blender, mix together the nutritional yeast, tofu, cornstarch, mustard, herbs, garlic powder, and red pepper flakes. Blend the ingredients together until the mixture is smooth. If necessary, scrape the sides.

Cook the vegetables first, then add the sauce from the blender to the cooked vegetables.

Fill a spring foam pan halfway with the frittata mixture and bake. Bake for 45 minutes at 350°F.

Sliced avocado can be added to the frittata for extra creaminess.

Chapter 5

Tomato Cups with Baked Eggs

This recipe is ideal if you want something quick and easy to prepare. Indeed, the simplicity of this recipe makes it one of the best ways to try eggs from cage-free, organically fed chickens. This is a simple breakfast recipe that you can add to your menu. This dish can also be served as a side dish for lunch or dinner. This is a quick and easy breakfast recipe that is healthy and flavorful.

Ingredients

6 tblsp. tomato

1 to 2 teaspoons extra virgin olive oil

salt and black pepper 1 teaspoon dried oregano, 6 ounces fat-free mild cheddar cheese, 1/3 cup fresh parsley Directions for Making Food

Preheat the oven to 350 degrees Fahrenheit.

Grease a muffin tin and set it aside with some cooking spray.

The tomatoes' tops should be cut off and removed. Removing the insides of the tomatoes with a melon baller Set them aside to be used in other ways.

Cut the tomatoes in half and place them cut side down on a paper towel or plate. Allow for a ten-minute rest period.

Cut side up, place the tomatoes in the muffin tin. Toss the tomatoes with olive oil.

Using pepper and salt, season the tomatoes. To the tomatoes, you can also add a pinch of dried oregano.

12 minutes in the oven, the tomatoes Remove them from the broiler and crack an egg into each of them from then on.

Bake for another 15 minutes, or until the eggs start to set. Prepare the egg yolks for more than five minutes if you don't need them runny or delicate. 9. Sprinkle the cheddar cheese on top of the eggs and heat until the cheese is melted.

10. Take the substance out of the oven and set it aside for two minutes to cool. After they've rested, garnish with parsley before serving.

5. Smoky Butternut Squash Breakfast Hash with Apples, Tofu, and

Hash is a dish made with diced or chopped meat, spices, and potatoes. All of these ingredients are combined and cooked with additional ingredients, such as onions. Sweet potatoes are replaced with butternut squash in this recipe. Apples and onions are a popular combination.

This recipe cooks the squash slightly hands-off rather than in a skillet, resulting in crispier squash. When the dish is done, you'll have a lovely autumnal breakfast dish on your hands. This dish is high in protein and can be modified by adding or changing the vegetables. Try rutabaga, collard greens, and parsnips, for example.

   2 tablespoons natural vegetable oil, such as refined avocado or grapeseed 1-1/4 pound butternut squash, peeled, seeded, and cubed 1-2 pieces of small apple

   8 oz. of tofu

   3 cups shaved Brussel sprouts, 3 tablespoons smoked paprika, 34 tablespoons low-sodium tamari or coconut amino, 1 tablespoon onion 1-1/2 tablespoons apple cider vinegar

   salt and black pepper

   Optional hot sauce and whole grain toast

   Directions for Making Food

   Preheat the oven to 400°F and prepare the baking sheet by lining it with foil or other material. Toss the apple, squash, and one tablespoon of oil in a dish.

   Add the pepper and salt to the mixture on the baking sheet. Continue to broil the apple and squash for at least another 35 minutes, or until they are tender and crisp around the edges.

   Over a medium heat, pour the remaining oil into a deep and large skillet. Cook the tofu shapes, tamari/coconut aminos, and smoked paprika. As much as possible, ensure that you mix. Cook the Brussel sprouts until they are tender and crisp, about 10 minutes.

Crumble the apples and squash that have been simmering and add to the pot.

vinaigrettes Add pepper and salt to taste after blending and mixing all of the ingredients. Carry on with the vinegar in a similar manner.

You can serve the dish with hot sauce or whole grain toast once it's finished.

Chapter 6

Breakfast Fajitas on the Sheet Pan

B reakfast fajitas in sheet containers are regarded as one of the most delicious Pegan breakfast ideas. These fajitas are packed with onion, a variety of ringer peppers, perfectly prepared eggs, and other ingredients. The fact that everything is done on the sheet skillet means you don't need to use anything else is perhaps the most amazing aspect of this recipe. To make this recipe, simply chop the vegetables, season them, and bake them until soft.

  This dish is full of nutrients and supplements like lutein, Vitamin B12, and Vitamin E, in addition to being simple to prepare.

1 tablespoon Paprika, 1 teaspoon Cumin, 1-1/2 teaspoons Onion powder, 14 teaspoons Pepper and salt Red bell pepper, 1 thinly sliced Green bell pepper, 1 thinly sliced Orange bell

pepper, 1 thinly sliced Olive oil, 2 tablespoons Chili powder, 1 tablespoon Garlic, 3, minced Lime juice, 1 tablespoon Paprika, 1 teaspoon Cumin, 1-1/2 teaspoons Onion powder, 14 teaspoons Pepper and salt

Eggs, 1 peeled, seeded, halved, and sliced avocado Cilantro leaves, 14 cup, chopped

Directions for Making Food

Preheat the oven to 400 degrees Fahrenheit. In the meantime, lightly oil or spray the baking sheet.

Mix onion powder, paprika, cumin, garlic, lime juice, bean stew powder, and olive oil with all of the chime pepper variations on the baking sheet. Continue throwing until the mixture has reached the desired consistency; season to taste with salt and pepper.

3. Cook for 15 minutes, or until the meat is tender.

Take this mixture off the stove and divide it into six wells. Begin to crack the eggs, being careful not to break the yolk. Taste the dish and season it with salt and pepper as needed.

Return the mixture to the broiler and cook for another 10 minutes, or until the egg whites are firm.

Serve the dish immediately; depending on your preferences, you can top it with cilantro or avocado.

Salads and soups are some of the most popular dishes in the United States.

Some extraordinary Pegan plans for soups and mixed greens are:

1. Chicken and Vegetable Soup with Bone Broth

This is a tasty and healthy supporting soup that you should consume every 2-3 days. If you have influenza, a cold, or simply need to warm up during the colder months, this is the dish for you. There's a lot going on in this soup: chicken bones, garlic, turmeric, and shiitake mushrooms, all of which are high in nutrients.

Shiitake mushrooms are a force to be reckoned with when it comes to sustenance. They're also known as beta-glucans, which support and energize the growth of beneficial microscopic organisms in the intestines. Your immune system will improve and you will live a longer life if your stomach contains beneficial microscopic organisms.

3 pound bulb garlic, 6 cloves yellow onion, 1 sliced carrot, 3 chopped Shiitake mushroom, 1-1/2 cup or 12 sliced celery stalks, 2 chopped Turmeric, 1 inch, peeled and chopped 1 pack Peppercorns, 12 teaspoon Sea salt Water, 10 cups Fresh ginger, 1 inch, peeled and chopped (Optional) baby spinach Directions for Making Food

Start by combining all of the ingredients in a large pot, excluding the water.

Fill the pot with water until all of the ingredients are submerged but not spilling. Around ten cups of water should suffice.

Begin heating the ingredients, then cover and allow to simmer.

After 30 minutes, skim the top of the soup to remove any non-edibles that have risen to the surface.

Allow for a minimum of two hours and a maximum of six hours of simmering time in the pot.

Sift the soup once it's finished to remove the chicken and vegetables; additionally, the extra chicken meat can be used in other dishes. Using two sifters, sift the soup.

While the stock is being served, add the chicken meat, mushrooms, and carrots (optional).

Soup with Golden Beets and Potatoes on a Sheet Pan

This soup is perhaps the simplest to prepare. Simply prepare your preferred vegetables and place them in a pot to cool. Mix or stock can also be added. You don't have to stand over the oven mixing the pot and inhaling steam.

The best part about this dish is that you don't have to be a professional chef to make it. These vegetables should be cooked simply. Nonetheless, you must exercise caution so that the ingredients do not become overcooked.

2 pound peeled and chopped golden beets Avocado oil, 2 tablespoons Russet or Yukon gold potatoes, 2 large, peeled and cut Yellow onion, 2 peeled and chopped

4 cups water 4 peeled garlic cloves

1 table spoon lemon juice

As a garnish: Hearts made of hemp Sprouts

Radishes cut with fresh dill Cooking Directions for Avocado

Preheating the broiler to 400°F is required. To ensure that the beets heat up quickly, cut them into 12-inch pieces. Place them on a baking sheet, drizzle with oil, and toss to combine. Broil them for ten minutes, or until they are golden brown.

If they obscure or turn black, that's fine.

Prepare the potatoes by chopping them into 1-inch pieces while the beets cook. In addition, slash the onions.

Put them in a separate baking dish, along with the whole garlic cloves. Pour some oil on the table and cover it with a blanket. Add the second plate to the stove after the beets are finished. Presently,

Another 30 minutes of broiling the two plates is required.

Blend the vegetables and beets when they are soft. Similarly, toss in some pepper, salt, and water.

a similar concept Make sure to thoroughly mix the ingredients.

After that, squeeze some lemon juice over them and garnish with whatever you want.

5. Chicken Soup (Southwest)

This particular dish, also known as detoxifying southwest chicken soup, is a simple vegetable and chicken soup with a variety of detoxifying ingredients. You can eat this soup for a long time in a row to re-energize your stomach-related framework.

This soup is gluten-free, paleo, low-carb, and low-fat, and it works exactly as it should to cleanse your digestive system. Combination of

If you're looking for an enticing striking character, green chilies and flavors will enhance the type of vegetables and chicken you're using. This soup can sneak up on you in terms of flavor. You also don't have to be a Masterchef to make this delicious soup.

1-1/2 pound skinless and boneless chicken breasts 1 peeled and chopped large onion 4 minced garlic cloves Olive oil, 1 tablespoon green chilies

14.5 oz. roasted and crushed tomatoes 12 teaspoons turmeric, 3 quarters cumin, 3 quarters cumin

Carrots, 2-1/2 cups, sliced Cabbage, 4 cups, chopped Broccoli florets, 3 cups Crushed red pepper, 1 teaspoon Avocados, 2, peeled and diced salt and black pepper

Directions for Making Food

Add olive oil, garlic, and slashed onions to a large pot set over medium-high heat. Cook the mixture for five minutes, or until the fixings become delicate. In a large mixing bowl, combine the chicken bosoms, carrots, spices, stock, squashed tomatoes, green chilies, and salt.

Reduce the heat and simmer for 20 minutes. Make sure the chicken breasts are fully cooked. Remove the chicken and place it on a cutting board using a couple of utensils.

Toss in the broccoli and hacked cabbage and continue to cook until the broccoli is tender. Meanwhile, shred the bosoms and re-add them to the soup.

Add salt to taste once the broccoli has softened. When serving, toss in the avocado.

Salad Bowl of Quinoa Pegan

This pegan-friendly quinoa salad bowl is a tasty option. This dish has a lower carb count because it doesn't contain any grains. Quinoa has a high protein content due to its seed status. In addition, the vegetables are low in calories and do not contain any starch. This salad is a delicious light serving of mixed greens that is perfect for your lunchbox and pleasing to the eyes.

Soak the black beans overnight and pressure cook for four minutes. Also, make sure the steam is allowed to escape normally and the liquid is allowed to drain naturally. This liquid can be used as a stock or as a dough kneader.

Quinoa, 1 cup, cooked (for the salad)

12 cup cooked and drained black beans, 12 cup shredded cabbage, 12 cup shredded onion, 14 cup chopped cucumber, 12 cup baby spinach leaves

Dressing Ingredients

Black pepper

Lemon juice, 3 tablespoons Miso paste, 1 tablespoon

Directions for Making Food

To start with, you really want to wash and cook the quinoa. When done, put it to the side to cool down.

Collect the wide range of various elements for the plate of mixed greens; wash them appropriately and channel them.

Begin by slicing the cucumber and onions, as well as shredding the cabbage. Put them in a bowl and arrange them on different sides once they're done.

Add the dark beans to the bowl after they've been washed and drained.

Add the quinoa to the bowl and mix well.

Whisk the lemon juice, miso, salt, and pepper for the dressing. Add this dressing over the serving of mixed greens and prepare if desired.

Chapter 7

Buddha Bowl

This unconventional bowl is an extraordinary choice assuming you are searching for Pegan- based servings of mixed greens. This vegetable comprises of vegetables, quinoa, and eggs, which makes it an ideal formula assuming you are searching for something light and healthy.

   This salad doesn't contain handled fixings and added substances. These vegetables don't contain any starch.

Ingredients Button mushroom, 300 grams, sautéed Asparagus, 200 grams, sautéed Boiled eggs, 6 Quinoa, 1-1/2 cups, sautéed Red capsicum, 1 Zucchini, ½ Iceberg lettuce, 1 head Colored cabbage, ¼ cup, optional Onions, 2, chopped Garlic, 8 cloves, minced Red chili powder, ½ teaspoon
   Salt Cherry tomatoes, 15-20 Carrot sticks, 1 cup Pumpkin seeds

Directions for Making Food

First, you need to gather the mushrooms and water into a single unit to wash away the coarseness. Add the eggs to the water to

bubble and furthermore add salt. In another skillet, add quinoa and water and begin bowling it as well.

Start cutting the vegetables. Hack the onions and mince the garlic. Cut and dry the mushrooms in an even size. Strip the asparagus and hack the broccoli.

Once the eggs are bubbled, strip and set them aside.

Add the salt and quinoa to the bubbling water and blend it well. Guarantee the fire is on the low setting.

Add the onions, garlic, and salt to the mushroom.

Additionally, add some stew powder and set it aside.

Drain the eggs and add water and broccoli to a similar container; continue to steam the broccoli until it becomes edible.

Take a pot and add olive oil and garlic. Continue to broil this blend until the crude smell vanishes. Add the asparagus now and continue sautéing it until it is done.

Add the other onions, garlic, and oil and sauté. Add the cooled quinoa to the mix.

Add lettuce leaves, sautéed quinoa, eggs, vegetables, and mushrooms to serve.

Snacks and Starters

Some incredible tidbits and starters would include:

1. Sautéed Collard Green Omelet

You can now enjoy your collard greens by converting them into a delicious snack. This dish has been rated as one of the best and can easily make your tongue shout out. It does not matter how you have prepared the collard. The point of this dish is to have well-seasoned and savory cooked greens. With the help of these greens, bacon or American pancetta, and some chipotle sauce, this omelet is definitely something to remember.

Ingredients

Butter, 3 tablespoons

American pancetta or Double smoked bacon, ½-inch or 4 oz, respectively

Hearty greens like beet greens, dandelion greens, mustard greens, collard greens, 1 lb, stems removed

Water, chicken stock or vegetable stock, ¼ cup Chipotle hot sauce

salt and black pepper Chardonnay vinegar Eggs, 4 Parsley, finely chopped

Directions for Making Food

On a nonstick dish, add the spread and let it liquefy. Then, add the pancetta and cook it until it

is fresh and brilliant brown; it ought not require over ten minutes. Also, the fats should be rendered.

Add the vinegar, hot sauce, and the greens and cook for around five minutes, or until the greens start to wilt.

Season with pepper and salt and add some stock assuming the greens begin drying prior to getting soft.

Add spread to one more nonstick skillet and hotness it over medium fire. The spread requirements to begin shimmering.

Whisk the eggs in a bowl until it has a cushioned and light consistency. Add a few pepper and salt as per taste. Empty the eggs into the butter.

Let the eggs cook; once done, drive the eggs into the focal point of the skillet with an elastic spatula to allow the fluid egg to cook. Continue to rehash until there is no fluid left.

Place the greens under the focal point of the egg and roll it in a round and hollow shape. Season it with pepper and salt and topping the dish with parsley.

2. Pan-Seared Salmon with Apple Salad and Kale

While this dish may look very fancy, it is very easy to prepare and cook. You can easily have it as a mid-day or evening snack. The salmon does not take more than ten minutes to cook in the skillet. Additionally, the flavors of the crunchy kale simply meld into the fish. All you need to do is add the wholewheat roll and the dish is ready to serve. This dish is sweet, tangy, and crunchy.

Ingredients

Salmon fillets, 4 Fresh lemon juice, 3 tablespoons Olive oil, 3 tablespoons

Salt and pepper

Kale, 1 bunch, leaves thinly sliced and ribs removed Dates, ¼ cup Honeycrisp apple, 1 Pecorino, ¼ cup, finely grated

Slivered almonds, 3 tablespoons, toasted Whole wheat dinner rolls, 4

Directions for Making Food

Before cooking, get the salmon filets to room temperature.

In a container, whisk together the salt, olive oil, and lemon juice. Add the kale and throw it to blend it appropriately. Allow it to represent ten minutes.

Meanwhile, cut the apples into matchsticks and dates into bits. Add the almonds, cheddar, apples, and dates to the kale. Season the blend with pepper, throw it and set it aside.

Sprinkle a few peppers and salt into the salmon. Take a nonstick skillet and add the excess oil over medium fire. Place them skinside up salmon into the container and raise the hotness. Cook for around four minutes or when the salmon becomes brilliant brown on one side.

Flip the salmon and continue to cook it for an additional three minutes or until it becomes firm.

Place the salmon, rolls, and salad on a plate to serve.

3. Grilled Vegetables with Creamy Cilantro Dip

If you like grilled vegetables, then this is the perfect recipe for you. This dish can also be consumed by people that want to lose weight. This dish is glutenfree and does not contain any dairy. The vegetables are only marinated in a dressing that is made with green chilies, ginger, garlic, and olive oil. As for the goat cheese, it is optional.

Ingredients Button mushrooms, 7-8 pieces Red onion, 1 cup, cubed Bell peppers, 1 cup, cubed Cherry tomatoes, 7-8 Zucchini, ½ cup, thickly sliced Green chilies, 1-2 Ginger, 1 piece Garlic cloves, 5-6 Mint leaves, 1 teaspoon Olive oil, 1-2 tablespoon Raw agave or any other plant-based sweetener, ½ teaspoon Red chili powder, 1 teaspoon Cumin powder, ½ teaspoon Dry mango powder, ½ teaspoon Goat cheese Turmeric powder, ¼ teaspoon Salt, as per taste

For the avocado cilantro dip:

Avocado, 1 Fresh cilantro, 1 cup Lemon juice, 1 tablespoon Garlic cloves, 1-2 Green chilies, 1-2 Salt Cooking Instructions

Take the mushrooms and wash and pat them. Assuming they are large, cut them into more modest pieces. Take the ginger, garlic, and green chilies and add them to a mortar. Continue to crush them until they become smooth. Rather than green chilies, you can likewise utilize new mint leaves.

Take oil, flavor powders, sugar, glue, goat cheddar, and lemon juice. Add and mix them well.

Cut the vegetables into 3D shapes and marinate them into this blend. Utilize your hands for this.

Cover the bowl with a top or stick film. Save it in the fridge for one hour.

Once 60 minutes, barbecue the vegetables on all sides. In the case of utilizing the stove, preheat the broiler to 200°F and barbecue the vegetables for 10 minutes. Put the vegetables to the side once done.

Now, you can begin making the avocado and cilantro plunge. Begin by adding the fixings to the chopper or blender and continue to mix it until it has a smooth consistency.

Serve the vegetables with this dip.

4. Mexican Roasted Cauliflower

Most individuals would think about the Mexican simmered cauliflower as probably the best starter, particularly to follow a Pegan diet. These cauliflower florets are thrown in tasty flavors and simmered until they are caramelized and fresh. This dish can be presented with red onions, cilantro, and lime juice. This dish is vegetarian and gluten-free.

However, there are some precautions that you definitely need to take. For instance, the cauliflower florets will get mushy and soft if the oven is not hot enough; this means that the final dish will not be caramelized and crisp. Also, you need to ensure that the baking pan is not over- crowded; if this happens, the florets will steam even before it starts to crisp up.

Ingredients Cauliflower head, 1 large, cut into florets Avocado oil, 2 tablespoons Chili powder, 1 teaspoon Onion powder, ½ teaspoon Garlic powder, ½ teaspoon Cumin, ¼ teaspoon Salt, ¾ teaspoon Cilantro, ¼ cup Black pepper, ¼ teaspoon Red and

green onion, ¼ cup, diced Avocado, ½, sliced Lime wedges, 3
Cooking Instructions

Start by preheating the broiler to 425°F. Then, add the cauliflower florets with pepper, salt, cumin, onion powder, garlic powder, bean stew powder, and avocado oil. Blend the fixings properly.

Line the baking plate with material paper and spread the cauliflowers equitably. Cook for

around 20 minutes.

Remove from the stove and flip the cauliflower. Cook the Remove from the stove and flip the cauliflower. Cook the 12 minutes.

Remove the cauliflower from the stove and trimming them. You can serve the cauliflowers with avocado, lime wedges, onion, or potentially new cilantro.

Chapter 8

Caveman Chicken And Vegetable Roast

This stone age man chicken and vegetable meal is viewed as a flavorful sheet skillet feast that can be eaten by your loved ones. Notwithstanding you are counting calories or not, this dish is very heavenly and simple to cook.

The simmered vegetables are an ideal supplement to the chicken drumsticks. When joined together, they make for a simple and scrumptious weeknight dinner. The vegetables in this meal comprise of parsnips, onion, potato, and carrots.

These veggies are simmered alongside the garlic cloves and the chicken. The flavoring blend comprises of standard kitchen staples like ground dark pepper, salt, and dried thyme leaves.

Roasting the concentrates of the vegetables removes their pleasantness and makes them extremely delicate as well.

You additionally have the decision to prepare the dish with different sorts of flavors and spices. This is an incredible dish since it tends to be put together and doesn't need a ton of work. You should simply add the fixings together and let your stove wrap up of the work.

Ingredients Onions, 1, peeled and cut Garlic, 12 cloves Russet potato, 1 Parsnip, 1 Baby carrots, 1 cup Chicken drumsticks, 1-1/2 pounds, skin on

Olive oil, ¼ cup Apple cider vinegar, 1 tablespoon Dried thyme leaves, 1 teaspoon Salt, 1-1/2 teaspoons

Ground black pepper, ½ teaspoons

Directions for Making Food

Start by preheating the broiler to 400°F. Join every one of the fixings on a huge rimmed baking sheet. Throw and blend properly.

Place the combination in the broiler and dish it until the vegetables are delicate and the chicken is cooked through, or for about an hour.

In the halfway, make sure to mix. Serve the dish immediately.

6. Prosciutto Wrapped Asparagus

There is no question that asparagus and prosciutto are a paradise made match. The hearty and nutty kind of the asparagus lances must be supplemented by the freshness and pungency of the ham. They can be cooked in a broiler under a barbecue, seared, or barbecued on a grill. This dish is an incredible decision for engaging visitors. It can likewise be filled in as a starter dish for a party. You can likewise dunk these sticks in delicate bubbled eggs, rather than the customary toasted bread.

While this dish is extremely simple to make, you need to be careful as well. Always ensure that the prosciutto is of good quality and paper-thin. It is suggested that you pre-wrap the asparagus with the prosciutto before the arrival of your guests.

Ingredients Olive oil Prosciutto strips/slices, 6 Asparagus spears, 12 Cooking Instructions

Wash the asparagus well and chop 2-cm off the ends. Cut the prosciutto into 12 equal slices.

Arrange the prosciutto strips on a hacking board at a 45-degree angle. Place the asparagus directly across from the highest point of the prosciutto.

The asparagus tip and the bottom section of the meat strip should be on the same line. Fold the prosciutto bottom half around the asparagus stick to secure the meat.

Begin moving the asparagus vertically from here. The prosciutto strip will cover the whole lance from the base up since it is at a 45-degree angle. It makes no difference whether it covers the whole asparagus.

Fill a griddle halfway with oil and wait until it's smoking. Fry the asparagus wrapped in prosciutto for a few minutes, or until the prosciutto is crisp and golden.

Chapter 9

Lettuce Cups with Thai Chicken

One of today's most excellent solid meals is the Thai chicken lettuce cup. Because of the lime and other spices, this meal, also known as LarbGai, may be produced quickly and with a variety of tastes. This dish is well-known in Asian countries due to its outstanding qualities.

This meal is a visual and gastronomic extravaganza. With the fresh mash of the lettuce and the heat from the aromatic spices, it has the perfect balance of heat, harshness, taste, and sweetness. These lettuce cups are about new tastes, much like diverse sorts of Thai culinary methods. Only a smidgeon of fish sauce and lime juice are used to make the sauce. Other aromatics such as lemongrass, shallot, garlic, and ginger, which are sautéed until the dish turns dazzling, provide a significant portion of the taste. Even before adding the chicken, fresh spices, and sauce, it starts to smell quite delicious at this point.

Ingredients

450g chopped chicken

de-seeded and coarsely chopped red chiles, 2 2 cloves minced garlic, 1 finely chopped lemongrass stalk, 1 inch grated ginger, 2 tablespoons lime juice

Mint leaves and fresh coriander Gem-shaped lettuce leaves Directions for Making Food

In a griddle or pan, pour the olive oil. Place the ginger in the pot.

Cook for 1 minute with the lemongrass, garlic, and bean stew.

Cook until the chicken is cooked through, about 10 minutes.

4 minutes more

Toss with a squeeze of lime and a pinch of fish sauce. Cook until all of the flavors have melded together.

Sprinkle thin bits of red bean stew, coriander, and more sliced mint over the mixture in the cleansed lettuce cups.

Entrees

If you're looking for some fantastic Pegan courses, have a look at the following list:

Greens with Turmeric in a Sauté

The majority of people are unaware of the health benefits of turmeric. Many others are unsure how to include it into their meal. Thankfully, this particular recipe is simple to prepare and includes turmeric.

We put turmeric in our smoothies. Perhaps its most appealing feature is that it has a bold taste that isn't overpowering, which is why even children like it. Turmeric may be used in a variety of meals, like this turmeric sautéed greens, in addition to smoothies.

Turmeric has been used for millennia and has a long history of use. It offers a variety of beneficial and natural qualities, including natural anti-inflammatory capabilities. You may get a lot of healing effects only by using turmeric in different foods.

1 tablespoon extra virgin olive oil, 3 minced garlic cloves 14 teaspoon water, 2 teaspoons fresh turmeric, 12 inch Swiss chard, spinach, or kale, 2 bunch each, thinly sliced Kosher salt

Directions for Making Food

Make sure you wash the greens well before chopping them. Mince them thinly once they've been washed and cleaned.

Add a couple tablespoons of oil to a large saucepan and heat it over medium heat.

Start by sautéing for a minute with salt and your favorite greens.

Pour the water into the pan and heat until the greens are just wilted, about 5 minutes.

Serve by transferring the mixture to a bowl.

Chapter 10

Sticky Chicken from Japan

The most flavorful dinner to prepare and make is probably Japanese sticky chicken. If you're looking for a quick, easy, and family-friendly recipe, this is it.

Chicken is one of today's most versatile protein sources, and it's also kid-friendly. In either event, it's all about how you're going to deal with it. This unusual meal has a spicy and sweet flavor that will make you drool and your fingers "licking nice."

This recipe is really adaptable, and you can easily swap out some of the ingredients to create something unique. Whether or not you can finish the whole meal in one sitting, the leftovers will be just as delicious as the main course. This chicken dish is often served with earthy colored rice and salad, making it an excellent summer supper.

Fresh ginger, 1 tablespoon Mirin, 14 cup Honey, 14 cup Low

sodium soy sauce, 14 cup Rice vinegar, 1 tablespoon Sesame oil, 1 tablespoon Togarashi spice mix, 1 teaspoon Skin-on chicken breasts, 2 bone-in chicken legs, 4 bone-in Scallions, 3 chopped

Directions for Making Food

Togarashi flavor mix, sesame oil, rice vinegar, soy sauce, honey, mirin, and ginger should all be whisked together in a baking dish or large zipper pack.

Continue turning the pieces as you add the chicken pieces from this combo. Leave the chicken in the marinade for an hour or overnight in the fridge.

Preheat the oven to 450 degrees Fahrenheit and add the marinated chicken.

Heat the chicken skin side up for 30 minutes or until golden brown.

Scatter scallions on top before serving.

Chapter 11

Scramble with Smoked Salmon

Salmon is said to be one of the greatest sources of omega-3 unsaturated fats, making it an excellent choice for you and your family. This protein-rich breakfast or dinner recipe is really easy to prepare. As an end-of-week casual breakfast for the whole family, you may also serve it with new organic goods, bagels, or freshly squeezed orange.

Cold smoked and hot smoked salmon are also available. The surface of cold smoked salmon is very rich and delicate since it is not heated. Hot smoked salmon, on the other hand, is cooked throughout the smoking process and hence has a strong flavor.

If you follow the instructions, making fried eggs should be a breeze. For your own health's sake, make sure the eggs aren't broken or dirty. Please check that no shells are broken into the eggs before breaking them into the dish. Prior to frying the eggs, it's advised that you lightly beat them.

Additionally, use just canola oil, which will give the meal a distinct taste.

We used hot smoked salmon to create this meal. Cold-smoked salmon, on the other hand, may be used; it will remain delicate and delicate. It is recommended that the meal be served right away for the greatest appearance and taste.

8 eggs, 4 chives, 4 tsp. Kosher salt, 12 tsp. Canola oil, 2 tsp. salmon, thinly sliced

Directions for Making Food

Two salmon chops should be set aside for garnishing; the remaining two should be cleaved into small pieces.

Season the eggs with salt and whisk them for certain chives.

Add the eggs to a preheated container. Continue scrambling the eggs, being careful not to overcook them.

Add the sliced salmon after the eggs have been cooked but not dried together. As soon as you remove the skillet from the burner, place it on a trivet.

Serve the eggs right away with the remaining chives and salmon.

4. Cauliflower Rice with Asian Flavours

Because of a variety of factors, this Asian cauliflower rice is a popular option for dinners. This meal, for example, has a vibrant hue. There are also many veggies in it. Of course, you may add whatever veggies you choose to this recipe; the option is yours.

Avocado oil, 1 teaspoon Eggs, 3 tablespoons Sesame oil, 1 tablespoon, roasted Avocado oil, 3 tablespoons Red onion, 1 tiny chopped ginger, 2 teaspoons 3 CUP RICED CAULIFLOWERS

8 oz. broccoli florets carrots (two) diced

Asparagus spears, 6, sliced into 1-inch chunks Crimini mushrooms, 6 oz. 12 cup cut snow peas 8 minced garlic cloves 1 diced red bell pepper 1 teaspoon Kosher salt 1 teaspoon onion powder 1 teaspoon sesame seeds

Onions that are green

Sauce ingredients:

1 tablespoon Rice vinegar, 1 tablespoon Fish sauce, 1 teaspoon Coconut aminos, 1/3 cup Toasted sesame oil

Directions for Making Food

Fill a sauté pot halfway with avocado oil and set aside to heat up. In the meanwhile, whisk the eggs and pour them into the heated skillet. Cook the eggs until they are just soft, then remove them and store them. To get rid of any leftover eggs, thoroughly clean the container.

Warm the remaining avocado oil and sesame oil in the skillet. Sauté the chopped onion for five minutes, or until it is soft. Mix for another minute after adding the minced garlic.

Cook until the asparagus, mushrooms, carrots, broccoli, and riced cauliflower are soft. Cook thoroughly with the remaining ingredients, including pepper, salt, and garlic. You may start making the sauce while the veggies and rice are cooking. To make the sauce, combine all of the ingredients in a large mixing bowl. Combine the rice and veggies with the sauce and reduce the heat.

Add the fried eggs to the overall mish-mash after the sauce is completely submerged. Toss with sesame seeds and green onions right away.

Chapter 12

Caramelized Vegetables with Lemon Roasted Chicken

For a variety of reasons, this lemon broiled chicken with caramelized veggies is a true dinner dish. Broil the ingredients and you're done! Your scrumptious dinner is ready to be served. It's likely the finest chicken meal you'll ever make.

Even if there are leftovers, the chicken pieces will be more delicious than before since the tastes will have been combined more thoroughly and the chicken will remain juicy and moist under the skin. The acidic taste of simmering lemons can't be avoided, of course.

5 pound chicken, 1 lemon juice, 1 lemon (do not discard), 5 pound chicken 6 peeled and whole garlic cloves 20 sprigs fresh thyme, split

5 sprigs of fresh parsley 2 sprigs of fresh rosemary 3 tblsp. extra-virgin olive oil 12 teaspoon tarragon, 12 teaspoon

thyme, 12 teaspoon salt, 12 teaspoon pepper, 12 teaspoon tarragon Carrots, peeled and sliced into 1-inch chunks, 1 1/2 pound baby potatoes 1 finely chopped onion (large)

Season the veggies with salt and pepper.

Directions for Making Food

Preheat the oven to 400 degrees Fahrenheit. In the meanwhile, wash and rinse the chicken, remove the giblets from the cavity, wipe off the excess fat, and discard it. Toss the chicken with salt & pepper.

Lemon juice should be poured outwardly from the bird. Garlic cloves and lemon halves should also be added.

Place the garlic and lemon into the chicken, along with the rosemary, parsley, and young thyme branches.

The chicken should be rubbed with olive oil. In a small mixing bowl, combine the salt, pepper, thyme, and dry tarragon; massage the mixture over the chicken layer. Legs and wings should be tied together.

After an hour at room temperature, place the chicken on a large sheet dish.

In a large mixing basin, season the onions, carrots, potatoes, and remaining oil with salt and pepper. Arrange the veggies around the chicken and scatter the thyme branches.

Cook for 60 minutes under the broiler. Allow 15 minutes for cooling before cutting. Warm it up and serve.

Pork Tenderloin in Southern Style

Most people believe that cooking pork takes time, especially certain components like tenderloins; however, if you skip the marinating, this meal may be prepared in less than 20 minutes. The excess marinade may be cooked and served as a sauce, which is one of the greatest aspects of this meal. You may also serve the pork with sweet corn on the cob, mixed veggies, or garlic mashed potatoes as an option.

Ingredients

14 cup Bourbon, 14 cup Dijon mustard, 14 cup Brown sugar, 14 cup Olive oil, 3 tablespoon Fresh ginger, 1 tablespoon finely chopped Garlic cloves, 3, minced

Directions for Making Food

Combine the soy sauce, whiskey, earthy colored sugar, olive oil, and salt and pepper in a large mixing bowl.

Whisk together the mayonnaise and Dijon mustard in a bowl. Fill a glass container or a large zipper bag halfway with the mixture.

Pork tenderloins should be placed in a compartment or zipper bag.

Allow it to marinade for a couple of hours or overnight.

Preheat the burner on high heat and keep the meshes greased on the day you'll be cooking the pork.

Remove the pork from the holder or bag and cook it for 14 to 15 minutes on the grill. Turn it halfway once the internal temperature reaches 140°F. The rest of the marinade should be kept in the fridge.

Allow the pork to rest for a few minutes after removing it from the grill. Cook for 10 minutes while the meat is being rehydrated.

Depending on your preferences, slice the tenderloin and serve with the marinating sauce.

Olives with Lemon-Spiced Chicken

Chicken, as previously said, is considered one of the most important sources of protein in today's world. Chicken may be used in a variety of cuisines. One of the delectable options is this seasoned chicken with olives and lemon.

This meal hails from Morocco's mountainous area, but you don't need to visit there to enjoy it. It's really easy to make and only takes around 20 minutes to prepare. Depending on your taste and preferences, you may substitute other veggies and seasonings.

Ingredients

Saffron threads, 14 teaspoon crushed Garlic, 5 cloves, coarsely chopped 12 teaspoon ground ginger

12 teaspoon Turmeric, 12 teaspoon Sweet paprika, 1 teaspoon Ground cumin

black pepper, salt 1 cut chicken into 8-10 pieces

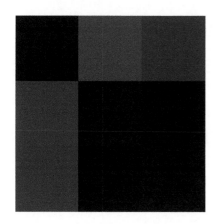

2 teaspoons of extra virgin olive oil

Calamata olives, 8, pitted and halved Onions, 3 thinly sliced Cinnamon stick, 1 8 pitted and halved green olives, crack

1 or 3 small or large preserved lemons 1 cup chicken stock; 12 lemon juice; 1 tablespoon chopped flat-leaf parsley

Directions for Making Food

In a mixing basin, whisk together the turmeric, cumin, paprika, ginger, saffron, and garlic. If you're not using real chicken, season it with salt as well. Combine the ingredients and apply to the chicken layer, cover, and marinate for 2-3 hours in the refrigerator.

Heat up some oil in a skillet. Cook for 15 minutes with a few onions added in. If you're using a tagine, transfer the mixture to it instead of leaving it in the skillet. Place the cinnamon stick in the mixture.

Remove the chicken from the cooler and combine it with the onions in the skillet. The olives should also be dispersed.

Remove the lemon mash and chop the skin into strips, then combine with the chicken. Combine the lemon juice and stock in the same way.

The skillet or tagine should be covered. Cook for 30 minutes on low heat, or until the chicken is done. Disperse the parsley on top of the dish before serving.

Sides Some of the most amazing Pegan sides have the following plans:

1. Almond Dip in Raw State

If you're searching for a Pegan hummus, this easy and delectable raw almond dip is a fantastic option. When these almonds are combined, a creamy and delectable spread is created. It's naturally gluten-free, vegan, low-carbohydrate, and raw, making it a fantastic choice for a large party.

There are a few of reasons why this almond plunge is a superior option for a healthy lifestyle. Almonds are rich in vitamins and nutrients and help to protect cells from oxidative stress. Vitamin B2, copper, manganese, and magnesium are also abundant.

It's best if the almonds are soaked beforehand. It also eliminates phytic acid molecules, which bond with minerals like as calcium, zinc, and iron, making them less accessible to the body. Soak them for at least six hours, but 12 hours is preferable.

1 cup soaking Extra virgin olive oil, 14 cup raw tahini, 14 cup water, 3/4 cup garlic, 2 cloves Lemon juice, 14 cup Salt, 12 teaspoon pepper crushed, 12 teaspoon cumin, 14 teaspoon turmeric powder, 3/4 teaspoon parsley, 14 cup, optional Directions for Making Food

To begin, soak the almonds for at least six hours; 12 hours is best. Make sure the almonds are completely dry before you use them.

In a blender, combine all of the ingredients and blend until smooth. Taste and adjust the flavoring as needed. If you want to add flavor and color, parsley is a great choice.

The hummus goes well with a variety of foods.

2. Zucchini Tortillas/Rotis (vegan)

If you're looking for dairy-free and low-carb sides, these vegan rotis/tortillas are the way to go. This dish is simple to prepare and allergy-free. They can also be prepared ahead of time and frozen for use the next day; simply reheat and serve.

Zucchini is a nutritious vegetable, as most of us already know. There aren't many carbohydrates in it. Almond flour, nutritional yeast, psyllium husk, and chia seeds are just a few of the other vegan ingredients in this dish. You can make the rotis/tortillas with either blanched almond flour or coconut flour.

Ingredients

3 grated Zucchini, 1 tablespoon coarsely powdered Psyllium husk, 2 tablespoon Nutritional yeast, 14 cup blanched almond flour, 2 tablespoon seasonings

Directions for Making Food 1. Wipe the zucchini clean after washing and drying it. Use a food processor or a box grater to grind the zucchini.

Fill a flavor or espresso processor halfway with chia seeds. Add psyllium husks to the mix when grinding.

In a large mixing bowl, combine the chia seeds powder, zucchini powder, psyllium husk, and salt and pepper. Also, don't forget to include the probiotic yeast. To set up the dough, thoroughly blend and consolidate.

Add some almond flour to help the batter set up. Allow ten minutes for the combination.

The rotis/tortillas can now be baked. Preheat the oven to 350 degrees Fahrenheit.

Lightly grease a baking sheet. Begin making a chunk of batter with a small portion of the batter.

To make slender plates for roti or tortillas, flatten the ball on a baking sheet.

Bake for ten minutes on both sides for each roti/tortilla. The tortillas will be cooked to a pleasant crispness after 20 minutes, with slightly brown edges.

3. Lemon Kale and White Beans with Sweet Potatoes

This yam with lemony kale and white beans makes an excellent dinner side dish. This side dish can be made quickly and easily without any preparation. It can also be used as a mixing bowl for mixed greens. Kale and yams are obviously nutritious.

On the lookout for the most expensive vegetables. This dish, in any case, is well worth the price.

You don't gain weight by eating low-calorie dishes. If you're feeling particularly energetic, you can make this dish with tofu or chicken and more pumpkin seeds. You will be pleasantly surprised by the flavor of this dish.

4 medium/large sweet potatoes 1 tablespoon optional olive oil Onion or shallots 1 to 2 cloves minced garlic, chopped

1 teaspoon of sea salt, 1 to 12 teaspoons lemon zest

1 bunch chopped kale with thick stems removed (alternatively, you can also use spinach, chard, baby kale, collards, etc.)

one can of cannellini beans

Optional: 1-112 teaspoon crushed red pepper flakes a squeeze of lemon

Pumpkin seeds with toasted tamari

Directions for Making Food

Preheat the stove to 350 degrees Fahrenheit. Meanwhile, wash and dry the potatoes, and prick the main with a fork a few times.

a fork as a utensil

Pre-heat a sauté dish; add the oil and the shallots and cook for two minutes.

Stir in the lemon zest, garlic, and salt for one minute more.

Cook an additional three minutes after adding the red pepper drops, beans, and kale. Season with a squeeze of lemon and a pinch of salt.

Allow the yams to cool after removing the skillet. Sprinkle the pumpkin seeds on top of the bean and kale mixture.

Vegetable Pizza with a Spiralized Sweet Potato Crust

This is a delectable vegetable-based pizza. The exterior is made up of perfectly spiralized potatoes.

Depending on your taste and preferences, you can also add a variety of vegetables to the top.

This is a vegetarian pizza that will redefine the term. Grain-free, paleo, vegan, and gluten-free, this dish is nutritious and filling. It's a unique take on a classic pizza night.

Ingredients: 1 spiralized sweet potato, 3 quartered large Brussels sprouts, 3 flax eggs, 2 baby radishes, 3 sliced 1-2 tablespoons Nutritional Yeast

Sauce ingredients:

12 teaspoon Dried oregano, 1 teaspoon Onion powder, 12 teaspoon Dried basil, 12 teaspoon Dried marjoram, 12 teaspoon Black Pepper, 14 teaspoon Cooking Instructions Unsalted tomato paste, 2 tablespoon minced garlic, 12 teaspoon Dried oregano, 1 teaspoon Onion powder, 12 teaspoon Dried basil, 12 teaspoon Dried marjoram, 12 teaspoon

Preheat the stove to 450°F to start the cooking process. Use your hands to combine the spiralized yam and flax egg.

In a small mixing bowl, combine all of the sauce's components.

Place the potato in the center of a greased baking dish, Silpat-lined baking sheet, or cast-iron skillet. Make sure the potatoes are shaped in a circular pattern.

With the help of a spoon, spread the sauce on the pizza's outer edge. Sprinkle some dietary yeast on top of the vegetables in the next layer.

Cook for 15 minutes after placing the pizza on the stove. To serve, remove the spatula from the plate with a spatula.

Desserts

Pegan dessert recipes include the following:

Apple Crisp from Pegan

Natural products such as apples, pumpkins, and pomegranates are considered to be at their peak during the fall season. You can make a delicious Pegan apple fresh with the help of apples, which is a healthy twist on the traditional apple fresh dish. This recipe is packed with healthy, whole ingredients that don't contain any sugar substitutes. A good pastry recipe will allow you to enjoy a sweet treat while also including some healthy ingredients such as gluten-free oats, grass-fed ghee, and apples.

Most people enjoy apples for a variety of reasons. These fruits are well-known for their dietary value. The fact that apples contain both soluble and insoluble fiber, which is essential for gut health, is one of their most distinguishing features. Apple fiber feeds the gut's short-chain fatty acids, which aids energy production in the large intestines.

Almond flour, 1/4 cup Gluten-free oats, 1/2 cup Apples, halved and cored

2 tablespoons of grass-fed ghee 14 cup of brown sugar

Directions for Making Food

Preheat the oven to 350 degrees Fahrenheit (180 degrees Celsius).

Place the apples in a baking dish, cut side up, cored side up.

In a small mixing bowl, combine the brown sugar, almond flour, and oats. Make a great connection.

Fill each divided apple with this mixture until it is completely filled.

Ghee should be drizzled over each apple/oat mixture.

Cook the apple/oat mixture on the stove for about 40 minutes, or until it is completely cooked and tender.

2. Paleo Brownies that are vegan and gluten-free

One of the quickest and easiest desserts to make is vegan paleo brownies. This is a delicious dessert that will leave you feeling completely guilt-free. You will not gain weight as a result of it. Depending on how long you keep them in the freezer, these brownies will be very crisp, with a deep chocolate flavor, and also very fudgy.

Ingredients

2-4 oz. maple syrup, 34 cup flax eggs, 12 cup cocoa powder, 12 cup unsweetened dark chocolate, melted coconut oil, 12 cup cocoa powder, 12 cup cocoa powder, 12 cup unsweetened dark chocolate, 2-4 oz. maple syrup (or actual eggs, if you are not vegan) 14 cup salt, 12 teaspoon vanilla, 1 teaspoon coconut flour, vanilla extract, 1 teaspoon coconut flour, 1 teaspoon coconut flour, 1 teaspoon coconut flour, 1 teaspoon coconut flour, 1 teaspoon coconut flour, 1 teaspoon coconut flour, 1 teaspoon coconut

Preheat the broiler to 350 degrees F and line a 12-pocket biscuit tin with a material paper liner.

In a medium-sized pot, melt the unsweetened chocolate, cocoa powder, and coconut oil. Continue whisking until the mixture is smooth and predictable.

Take the blend off the heat and stir in the maple syrup (or you can likewise utilize honey). The mixture will thicken over time.

Consolidate well with the vanilla and flax eggs.

Salt and coconut flour should be added at this point. Ensure that you keep consolidating until no dry pockets remain.

Fill the skillet halfway with the mixture and bake for 20 minutes.

Allow to cool before transferring to a cooler. However, there is no compelling reason to move something like a magma cake to the cooler if you are looking for it. The cooler is important for brownies because it determines consistency and texture. Smoothie made with strawberries and coconut

The best thing about this strawberry coconut smoothie is that it can be eaten for breakfast or as a dessert. This is a nutritious breakfast/dessert smoothie that will keep you energized. It will also aid digestion if you consume the smoothie after a heavy meal. The preparation is straightforward, and the smoothie will be ready in a matter of minutes.

1 cup coconut cream

1 cup frozen and sliced banana 2 cups frozen strawberries 1 teaspoon vanilla extract Vegan-friendly protein powder, 1 scoop vegan-friendly protein powder, 1 scoop vegan-friendly protein powder, vegan-friendly protein powder, vegan-friendly protein powder, vegan-friendly protein powder, vegan-friendly protein powder, vegan-friendly protein powder, vegan-friendly protein powder, vegan-friendly protein powder, vegan-

Directions for Making Food

Mix in all of the fixings until the mixture is silky smooth.

Continue to add coconut milk until the mixture reaches your desired thickness.

With ice, serve.

Chapter 13

Whipped Coconut Cream on Pegan Pancakes

Flapjacks can be served as a breakfast food or as a dessert after dinner. These hotcakes are made with quality ingredients and are incredibly easy to prepare. Aside from the healthy ones, there are no unusual additions.

2 large eggs (for the pancakes)
  12 cup almond milk (unsweetened) 2 teaspoons of pure vanilla extract melted 14 cup coconut oil
  Optional: 3 tablespoons granulated monk fruit sweetener 12 cup baking powder, 1 teaspoon baking soda, 12 teaspoon sea salt, 14 teaspoon ground cardamom 2 teaspoons ground cinnamon
  12 teaspoon crushed cloves 12 teaspoon crushed nutmeg 14 teaspoon ground ginger Optional use of pure maple syrup To

make the whipped cream, combine the following ingredients in a mixing bowl and whisk until

14 oz. chilled coconut cream 1/3 cup powdered monk's fruit

Directions for Making Food

In a mixing bowl, whisk together the almond milk, egg, coconut oil, vanilla extract, and priest organic product sugar until completely combined and feathery. Squash the pecans and add them to the mixture.

In a separate bowl, sift together the almond flour, buckwheat, salt, baking powder, cardamom, cinnamon, nutmeg, and cloves. After that, switch to the wet mixture and keep mixing until all of the protuberances have vanished. Start by heating up a large skillet. Brush the dish with the excess coconut oil and empty some of the container when it is sufficiently hot.

the participants are involved in it Allow for two minutes on each side of the blend to cook. On both sides, make sure the hotcakes are firm and golden brown. For the remaining batter, repeat the cycle.

To make the whipped cream, cool a large mixing bowl first. Remove the strong cream segment from the coconut cream in the cooler. Add the powdered priest foods grown from the remaining ground cinnamon and blend until smooth. Two minutes later, blend again.

Whipped cream is served alongside the hotcakes. Cut figs and a sprinkling of maple syrup on top, if desired.